Risks Of Product Use

This content is not a substitute for direct, personal, professional medical care or diagnosis. None of the diet plans or exercises (including products and services) mentioned by Mindful Health LLC or from Danette May should be performed or otherwise used without clearance from your physician or healthcare provider. The information contained within is not intended to provide specific physical or mental health advice, or any other advice whatsoever, for any individual or company and should not be relied upon in that regard. We are not medical professionals and nothing herein should be misconstrued to mean otherwise.

There may be risks associated with participating in activities contained herein for people in poor health or with pre-existing physical or mental health conditions. Because these risks exist, you will not participate in such diet plans if you are in poor health or have a pre-existing mental or physical condition. If you choose to participate in this program, you do so of your own free will and accord, knowingly and voluntarily assuming all risks associated with such dietary activities. These risks may also exist for those who are currently in good health right now.

In addition, this program includes training on how to perform bodyweight exercises. If done with poor form, any exercise, including bodyweight exercise, may carry inherit risk. Please consult your doctor before starting any diet or exercise program. Meal plans are also included in this program. User assumes all risks inherent with cooking and preparing foods.

Generally Expected Results From Mindful Health LLC and Other Danette May Products

We work very hard to make sure our customers achieve the best results possible. However, as with most things, results are determined by the amount of effort put in.

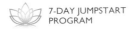

We've given you a clear blueprint to getting the best results possible, but in order to see results, you must follow the plan we give you each week. This program is designed to show you how to live a healthy lifestyle, and it's our goal to help you not only look better, but feel better on a daily basis. Results can't be guaranteed, because everyone is different and responds in a different way.

Testimonials Disclaimer

Testimonials found on a Mindful Health LLC website are results that have been forwarded to us by users of Danette May's programs, and may not reflect the typical purchaser's experience, may not apply to the average person and are not intended to represent or guarantee that anyone will achieve the same or similar results. If we have disclosed typical results based on information provided to us by a manufacturer or other reputable third party source, you should presume that the typical results as stated are more reliable than the testimonials and other examples found on our websites. However, you should always perform due diligence and not take such results at face value. We are not responsible for any errors or omissions in typical results information supplied to us by manufacturers or other reputable third parties. If a product or service is new, you understand that it may not have been available for purchase long enough to provide an accurate results history. Again, it is possible that even with perfect use of the program, you will not achieve the results described in testimonials. They are meant to be a showcase of the best results the program has produced, and should not be taken as the results a typical user will get.

Visit this link to view the full health disclaimer:
www.7djsdisclaimer.com

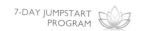

Table of Contents

The Program

Meet Danette	6
Ready for Mind Blowing Fat Loss Results?	9
Your 7-Day Plan Begins Now!	14
Creating Weekly Menus!	
For Women	18
For Men	41
Strength Training and HIIT	63
7-Day Fat Loss Fast Track Program	67
Weekly Workout Schedule	68
Sourcing Animal Products	72
The Superfoods	75
Why Water is Important for Fat Loss	84
The Gut Feeling	85
How To Combat Stress	87
Yoga & Meditations	91
Eating Organic	95
Congratulations!	97
Notes	98
Recommended Resources	100

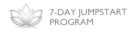

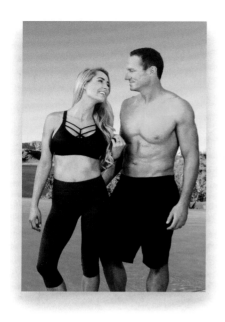

Hi there!

I wanted to take a moment to introduce myself and my husband, Craig, to share a bit about our journey. I think it's essential for you to get to know us better and understand why we've created this program for you!

We've discovered the power we have to heal our bodies through food, movement and shifting our mindset. We each came from very different backgrounds, yet through our own unique stories, have come together to SHARE our journey with others. Together we'll share the tools and lessons we've learned from our own transformations and share them with the world so that everyone can experience massive healing. Our mission on this planet is to empower others to RISE into radical self-love, and this all starts on the inside through balancing the hormones, decreasing inflammation in the organs and resetting your internal system.

In 2011 we founded Mindful Health, LLC where we've developed many programs to support over 2 million clients through body and mind transformation.

I am a world-renowned motivational speaker, #1 best-selling author of seven health and women empowerment books, former celebrity fitness trainer, proud wife, and mother of two loving daughters. I have also shared my unique, inspiring message on national TV, Access Hollywood, Hallmark Home and Family, CBS, and many others. Through sharing my message and developing my programs, I have helped transform the physical, mental, emotional, and spiritual lives of millions of people around the world.
I have worked with thousands of individuals worldwide who came to me as a last resort. They had tried ALL the fad "diets," pills and weight loss programs yet they did not see the results they desired. Why? Because their bodies were inflamed.

We all experience some levels of inflammation in our bodies, but with our current food additives, preservatives, food allergies, stress, toxins and sugar consumption, we see inflammation levels skyrocketing. Inflammation in the body can cause disruption to all of our major organs, inhibit digestion and absorption of our food, throw off our hormones and prevent us from losing that extra weight.

From many years of experience, we created this simple process with particular foods and healing movements that will clean out the gut and the organs allowing them to release stubborn body fat. Consuming non-inflammatory foods reduces acne, aches and pains in the joints, balances hormones, increases energy and so much more! You see, "clean eating" does not always work for everyone. Most of us need a deeper reset and jumpstart to our metabolism to truly see the results we desire.

This 7 Day Jump Start book was designed to educate you on inflammation within your body and share with you how to create a diet rich in healthy, yummy, non-inflammatory foods to heal your body and jump start your weight loss. I've included 3 full days of meal plans for both men and women to get you started. If you still need a little help, there's a bonus 7 day meal plan PDF that can be found here http://7dayjs.com/program/

I am so confident that my 7-Day Jumpstart WORKS, as the results will speak for themselves. We're so glad you are here, and are beyond excited for you to begin your transformation!

Welcome to YOUR 7-Day Jumpstart!

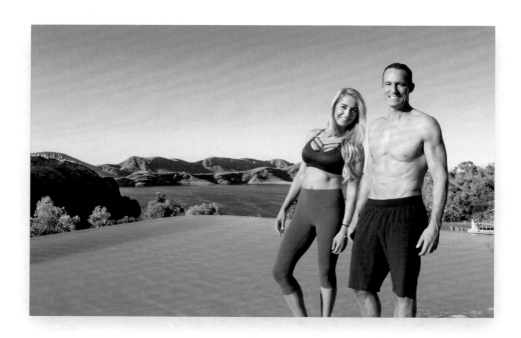

Ready for Mind Blowing Fat Loss Results?

Welcome to our 7-day rapid weight loss and body transformation program. Seven solid days of genuinely mind-blowing results if you follow the plan precisely as I have designed it! It is only seven days and will kick-start your body into becoming a fat burning machine! The incredible part about this program is that I'm giving you the opportunity to eat 6 times per day using our example meal plans and approved non-inflammatory foods. You will be eating healthy, high energy foods, and performing workouts that add strength, vitality, and vigor.

Other programs can give you extreme weight loss, by requiring you to consume very minimal calories, where you are left feeling "hangry!" hungry + angry! Or they may need you to take weight loss pills or drink nasty shakes that leave you hungry, empty and lethargic!

This program is so radically different than what you are used to, and I know you are going to love it and see LASTING results! The 7-Day Jumpstart focuses on eating whole, clean, anti-inflammatory foods that react in the body to burn up fat and shrink inflammation in your belly and thighs!

The combination of foods, the frequency (every 2-3 hours), and the right high energy, anti-inflammatory foods are what will give you surprising results with weight loss. Eating these super foods will also leave your skin, mind, and body feeling alive and vibrant.

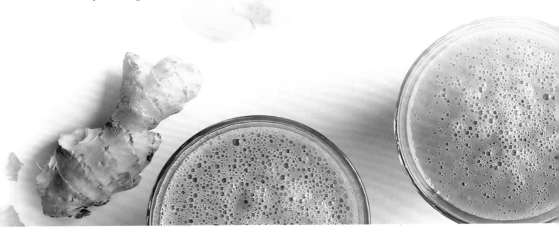

With the right foods fueling your body, in combination with multiple muscle engagement movements, you will add muscle while losing body fat in all the right places!

I created this program for hundreds of my clients to allow them to feel "HOPEFUL" again. It is never too late to lose weight and transform your body. Yes, you can even have more energy throughout the day and the bonus of increased libido!

Many of us use the excuse that we are not able to lose weight. We have tried countless weight loss pills, shakes, and programs, and then gain the weight right back, and sometimes more! You are going to LOVE my 7-Day Jumpstart and lose stubborn body fat, feel great while doing it, and keep it off LONG TERM.

Let's Get Started!

The fact that you signed up for my 7-Day Jumpstart proves you are ready to make a lasting change in your life. You've already learned what you need to know to make changes. Now it's time to begin the "preparation" for your jumpstart! Starting with a positive mindset is crucial for lasting results. I would like to take a minute and guide you through the preparatory steps necessary for success.

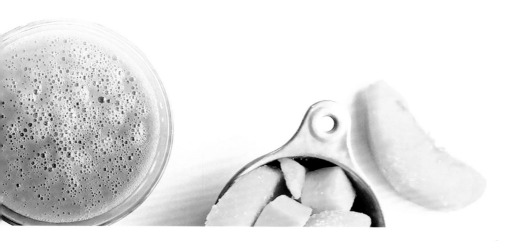

Step One

When you're preparing for a new meal plan, the following will help guide you. Write out your health and weight loss goals below.

How many pounds do you want to lose? This goal can go beyond what you will lose in 7 days.

_____

_____

_____

What is your ideal pant size?

_____

_____

How many inches do you want to lose around your waist?

_____

_____

Sleep goals:

_____

_____

_____

Energy goals:

_____

_____

Mood goals:

_____

_____

Write out your "WHY."

_____

_____

_____

_____

_____

_____

_____

Why are you doing this program?

_____

_____

_____

_____

_____

Why do you want to improve your health?

_____

_____

_____

_____

_____

Write down a detailed plan for what you'll do to make your diet changes. For example, what are you willing to give up to reach your goals? (alcohol, sugar, excuses, etc.)

_____

_____

_____

_____

_____

_____

What time will you do your exercises during the day?

_____

_____

What is your go-to plan when something unexpected happens that changes your planned routine?

_____

_____

_____

_____

_____

What will you do if someone tries to sabotage your success?

_____

_____

_____

_____

_____

Schedule your daily workouts ON your calendar to ensure you complete them. Block out 30-40 minutes a day for seven days to leave time for your warm up, workout and cool down.

Determine how you'll reward yourself once you have completed the 7-Day Jumpstart. Write it down, and post it where you will see it daily, so you have something to look forward to at the end of your seven days. It is important to celebrate and reward ourselves for our success. Otherwise, change can feel like a chore.

Clean out your kitchen! Go through your refrigerator and cupboards and get rid of anything that is not on the list of foods. You will have better control over what you consume when your house contains clean, healthy choices.

Your 7-Day Plan Begins Now!

Here is your list of non-inflammatory foods which were carefully chosen to support you in reducing inflammation in your body. I have eliminated all the guesswork, so all you need to do is stock your pantry and refrigerator with your favorites among this pre-approved list.

If there are some items on this list you haven't tried before, don't be nervous. Look at this as an opportunity to explore new foods as an experiment in finding just the right fit for you and your body.

Protein

Eggs
Fish (wild caught whenever possible)
Hummus
Kefir (plain*)
Lean chicken
Lean turkey
Legumes*
Nuts & seeds (raw & unsalted)
Organic plain Greek yogurt
Salmon*
Lean grass-fed beef
Steak
Chia seeds
Hemp seeds

Grains

Brown rice
Buckwheat*

Fats

Avocado
Extra virgin olive oil
Nuts* (raw & unsalted)
Coconut oil (unrefined)

Beverages

Water
Pomegranate juice
Black tea
White tea
Herbal tea
Red wine

Ezekiel bread
Old-fashioned oats (slow cook)
Quinoa

---

* Grains are also available in flour form.
* Caffeine and alcohol should be consumed in moderation, approximately 1 cup/day or less.

Fruit

Acai pulp juice
Apples
Blueberries
Cherries
Kiwi
Melons: cantaloupe/
watermelon
Oranges
Pears
Pink grapefruit
Plums
Pomegranates
Prunes
Raisins
Raspberries
Red grapes
Strawberries (or any berries)

Herbs

Bee pollen (supplement)
Chili peppers
Chives
Dill
Ginger
Lemon verbena
Orange mint
Oregano
Parsley
Rosemary
Sweet basil
Tarragon
Thyme
Turmeric

Vegetables

Any dark leafy vegetables
Beet greens
Beets
Broccoli florets
Brussels sprouts
Corn
Eggplant
Kale
Onions/leeks/scallions*
Red bell pepper
Spinach

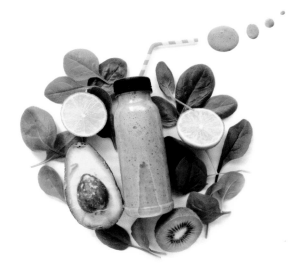

All foods with an asterisk (*) represent the 8 superfoods.

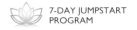

Women: Creating Your Weekly Menus!

Your success is only 7 days away!

Tips for success when implementing the 7-Day Jumpstart:

- Use ingredients from the list of approved non-inflammatory foods on pages 14-15 to create meals and snacks for your 7 day plan. If you still need a little help, we've created a bonus 7 day PDF with daily meal plans here http://7dayjs.com/program/

- Drink at least 1 gallon of water daily! You can flavor your water with fresh lemon & herbs.

- To jumpstart your metabolism make sure your first meal is within 1 hour of waking up. Eat each meal within 2-3 hours of one another.

- Use the link below to join my 30 day challenge - where I'll share a detailed step by step guide to detox your body, completely done-for-you 30 day meal plans that tells you what to eat and when, highly effective workouts, new meditations, deals, discounts and more.

30 Day Challenge: www.DanetteMay.com/start30dc

Embark on your journey of self-improvement by recording daily events to guide you towards a healthy lifestyle. Record them in a journal or right here. Below are a few ideas to get you started:

What did you eat?

_____

_____

How are you feeling?

_____

_____

_____

What was your workout?

_____

_____

_____

What made you smile today?

_____

_____

_____

Remind yourself of your "why." Write what is in YOUR heart!

_____

_____

_____

Weekly Menu For Women

Breakfast

- 3 ounces protein
- ¼ cup vegetables
- ½ cup carbs
- ¼ cup fruit

Snack

- 3 ounces protein
- ½ cup vegetables

Lunch

- 3 ounces protein
- ½ cup vegetables
- ½ cup fruit

Snack

- 3 ounces protein
- ¼ cup carbs
- 1 tablespoon healthy fats

Dinner

- 3 ounces protein
- ½ cup vegetables
- ½ cup carbs

Snack

- 3 ounces protein
- ¼ cup fruit

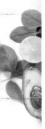

Day One Example Meal Plan For Women

Breakfast

EGGS & SPINACH
with Side of Oatmeal

Prep. time 15 minutes

Cook time 25 minutes

1 serving

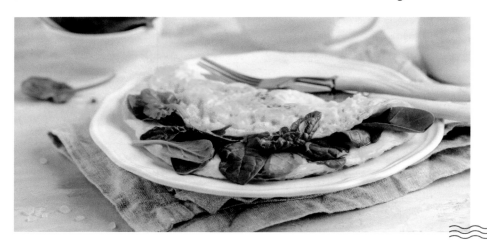

INGREDIENTS:

¼ cup spinach

1 tablespoon chopped onion

2 eggs

2 sprigs sweet basil

¼ cup oatmeal

¼ cup blueberries (or berries of choice)

1 teaspoon cinnamon

DIRECTIONS:

Coat skillet with non-stick cooking spray. Place 1/4 cup spinach & 1 tablespoon chopped onion in a skillet over medium heat, cook until wilted. Add 2 eggs, cook until done and top with sweet basil.

Cook ¼ cup oats according to the package. If you like creamier oatmeal, add water to desired consistency, top with berries and cinnamon.

7-DAY JUMPSTART PROGRAM

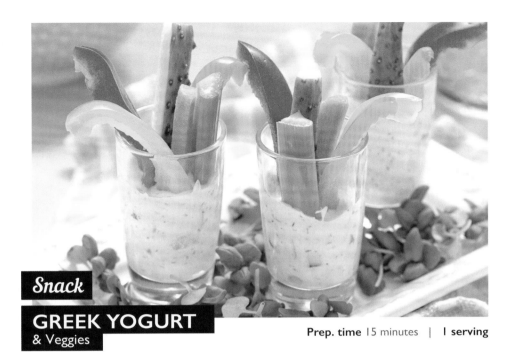

Snack

GREEK YOGURT
& Veggies

Prep. time 15 minutes | **1 serving**

INGREDIENTS:

½ cup plain Greek yogurt | crushed red pepper, to taste | rosemary, to taste | fresh dill, to taste | ½ cup sliced red pepper or vegetable of choice from approved list

DIRECTIONS:

Mix ½ cup plain Greek yogurt with crushed red pepper, rosemary & dill. Enjoy with ½ cup sliced red peppers or other vegetable of choice.

Lunch

GROUND TURKEY
with Warm Fruit Dessert

Prep. time 15 minutes

Cook time 25 minutes

1 serving

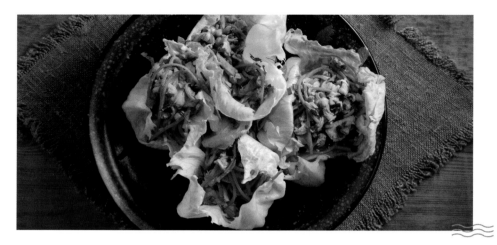

INGREDIENTS:

3 ounces ground turkey

1 teaspoon taco seasoning

½ cup of green lettuce of choice

fresh cilantro, chopped, to taste

½ c. apple or pear

pinch of cinnamon or nutmeg

DIRECTIONS:

Take 3 ounces ground turkey, cook in skillet until fully cooked, add 1 teaspoon taco seasoning. When evenly mixed, scoop turkey meat on ½ cup of greens and top with fresh cilantro.

Slice an apple or a pear, sprinkle with cinnamon or nutmeg. Place in pan and bake for 15 minutes in a 350°F. oven.

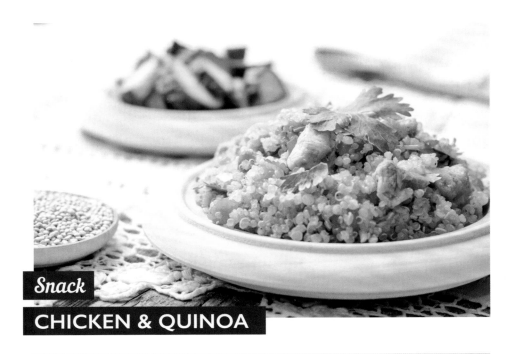

CHICKEN & QUINOA

Prep. time 15 minutes | **Cook time** 25 minutes | **1 serving**

INGREDIENTS:

¼ cup quinoa | 3 ounces cooked chicken, cubed | 1 tablespoon extra virgin olive oil | desired spices and herbs, to taste

DIRECTIONS:

Prepare a batch of quinoa according to packaging. Store in refrigerator and take out ¼ cup and add in 3 ounces cooked chicken breasts, cubed for a snack on the go. When ready to eat, drizzle 1 tablespoon of extra virgin olive oil and fresh spices and herbs.

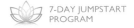

Dinner

SALMON & VEGGIES

Prep. time 15 minutes

Cook time 25 minutes

1 serving

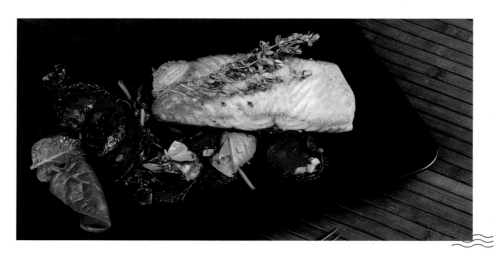

INGREDIENTS:

3 ounces wild caught salmon

½ cup beets or vegetables of choice, steamed

½ cup brown rice

juice from ½ of a lemon

black pepper, to taste

spice of choice (I like curry with this recipe), to taste

1 teaspoon extra virgin olive oil

DIRECTIONS:

Take 3 ounces salmon place in tin foil. Squeeze juice from ½ of a lemon on it and top with black pepper. Secure in tin foil and bake at 350 degrees for 30 minutes.

Cook brown rice according to package directions. Add any spice you would like.

Steam ½ cup of beets or vegetables, top with black pepper & 1 teaspoon extra virgin olive oil.

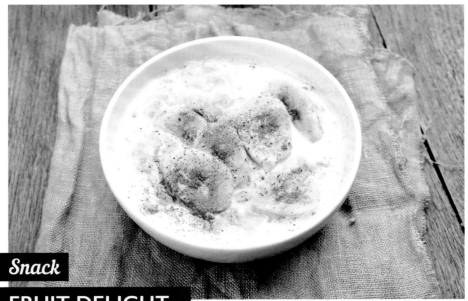

Snack

FRUIT DELIGHT

Prep. time 10 minutes | 1 **serving**

INGREDIENTS:

½ cup plain Greek yogurt | ¼ cup fruit of choice | cinnamon, to taste |
1 serving of stevia according to package. (choose a natural stevia)

DIRECTIONS:

Mix ½ cup plain Greek yogurt with ¼ cup fruit, sprinkle with cinnamon and
stevia. Enjoy!

Notes

7-DAY JUMPSTART
PROGRAM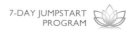

Breakfast

TOMATO AVOCADO
& Egg on Toast

Prep. time 15 minutes

Cook time 25 minutes

1 serving

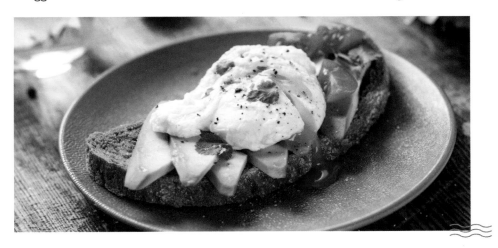

INGREDIENTS:

2-3 eggs

¼ avocado

½ roma tomato

1 slice of toasted Ezekiel bread

¼ c fruit of choice

DIRECTIONS:

Coat frying pan with non-stick cooking spray and fry eggs in a pan, over medium heat.

Toast Ezekiel bread, spread avocado on toast. Top with sliced tomato and fried eggs. Serve with ¼ c fruit of choice. Enjoy!

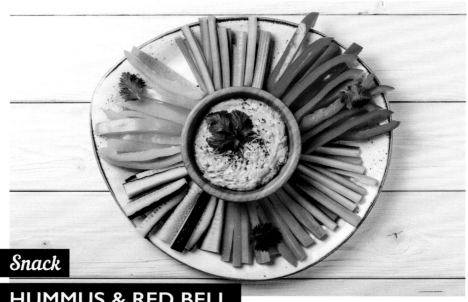

Snack

HUMMUS & RED BELL PEPPER SLICES

Prep. time 15 minutes | **1 serving**

INGREDIENTS:

1/2 cup garbanzo (chickpeas) beans rinsed & drained (reserve 1/8 - 1/4 cup of liquid) | 1 clove garlic | 1 tablespoon tahini | 1 teaspoon freshly squeezed lemon juice | 2 teaspoons extra virgin olive oil | 1/8 - 1/4 teaspoon cumin or chili powder (optional) | 1/4 teaspoon sea salt | pinch of black pepper | 1/2 cup sliced red peppers or vegetable of choice from approved list

DIRECTIONS:

Add garbanzo beans, garlic, tahini, lemon juice, extra virgin olive oil, sea salt, black pepper and 1/8 - 1/4 cup liquid from garbanzo beans. Add more if needed. Blend ingredients together until you get a thick, creamy mixture without any chunks. Eat hummus with 1/2 cup of sliced red pepper or other vegetable of choice. Enjoy!

Lunch

GREEK SALAD

Prep. time 15 minutes

1 serving

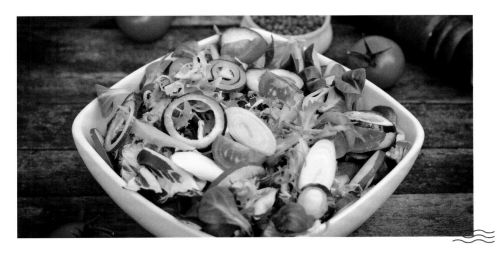

INGREDIENTS:

½ cup romaine lettuce, chopped

6 cherry tomatoes, halved

¼ cucumber, diced

1 tablespoon red onion, diced

1 tablespoon parsley, chopped

for vegetarians add 1 1/3 cups garbanzo (chickpeas) beans (rinsed & drained)

for meat eaters, add 3 ounces cooked chicken, cubed

DRESSING:

1 tablespoon extra virgin olive oil

1 tablespoon freshly squeezed lemon juice

DIRECTIONS:

Add all salad ingredients into a bowl. In a separate smaller bowl, mix dressing.

Drizzle dressing over salad and toss to mix.

Fruit and Nuts

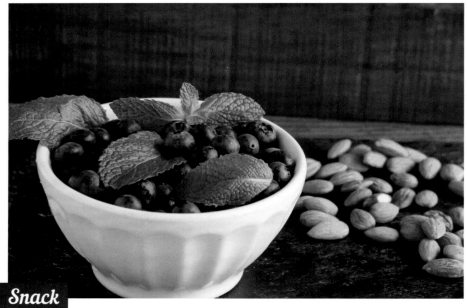

Snack

Prep. time 5 minutes | **1 serving**

INGREDIENTS:

¼ cup of raw almonds | ½ cup of berries (blueberries, raspberries or strawberries) | ½ c Greek yogurt

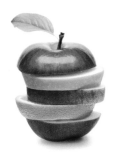

Do something today that your future self will thank you for.

7-DAY JUMPSTART
PROGRAM

Dinner

CHICKEN
with Broccoli & Rice

Prep. time 15 minutes

Cook time 25 minutes

1 serving

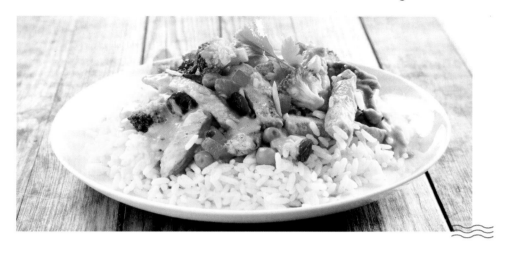

INGREDIENTS:

3 ounces chicken (grilled or cooked in pan)

½ cup broccoli florets

½ cup brown rice or quinoa

1 1/2 cups chicken or vegetable stock

1 teaspoon sea salt

1 teaspoon black pepper

1 tablespoon unrefined coconut oil

Note: juice from ½ of a lemon *(optional)*

DIRECTIONS:

Cook chicken in a pan with coconut oil until cooked through.

Steam broccoli florets. Cook rice or quinoa according to directions on package using chicken or vegetable stock instead of water to add flavor.

Season meal with sea salt, black pepper and any other preferred spices. Top with lemon juice *(optional)*.

Apples and Peanut Butter

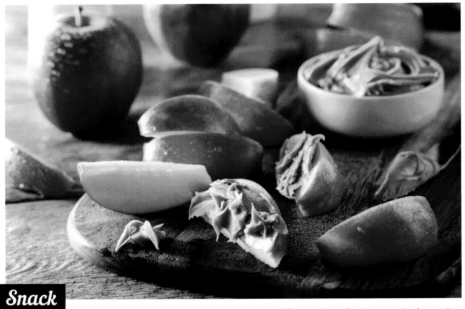

Snack

Prep. time 5 minutes | 1 serving

INGREDIENTS:

½ apple | 2 tablespoons raw peanut or almond butter

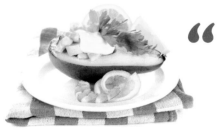

" *Every time you eat is an opportunity to nourish your body* "

Notes

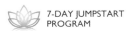

Day Three Example For Women

Breakfast

OAT BREAKFAST
with Fruit and Nuts

Prep. time 15 minutes	
1 serving	

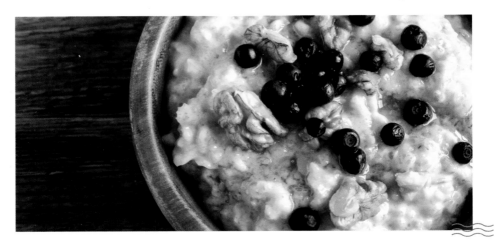

INGREDIENTS:

½ cup old-fashioned oats (slow cook)

¼ cup blueberries

¼ cup walnuts

pinch of cinnamon (optional)

¼ cup vegetables of choice from approved list.

½ c. Plain Greek Yogurt

DIRECTIONS:

Cook oats according to package. Top with berries, nuts and pinch of cinnamon if desired.

Eat with ¼ cup vegetables and ½ cup plain greek yogurt.

Eggs and Veggies

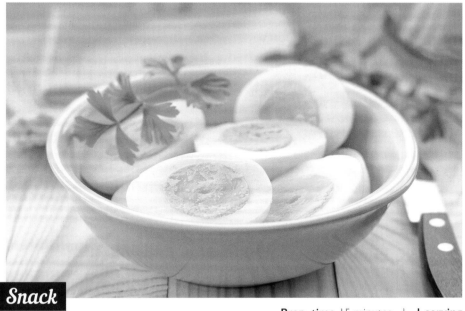

Snack

Prep. time 15 minutes | **1 serving**

INGREDIENTS:

2-3 hard boiled eggs | ½ cup red bell pepper slices

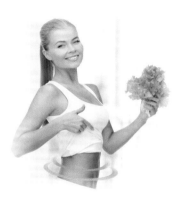

 Don't stop until you're proud

Lunch

QUINOA SALAD

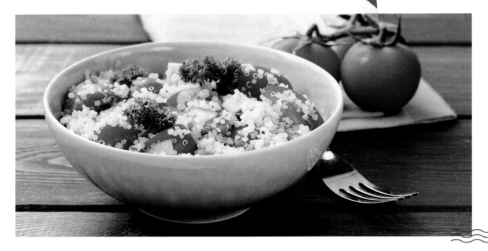

INGREDIENTS:

¼ cup cooked quinoa

¼ cucumber, diced

¼ cup walnuts, raw

¼ red bell pepper, diced

1 tablespoon extra virgin olive oil

1 tablespoon balsamic vinegar

3-4 sprigs of fresh parsley

sea salt and black pepper, to taste

½ cup of fruit from approved list

2 oz of cooked chicken (cubed)

DIRECTIONS:

Cook quinoa according to directions on the package and allow to cool. Add chicken, quinoa, cucumber, walnuts, and red pepper to a large mixing bowl. Add extra virgin olive oil, balsamic vinegar, salt and black pepper. Toss to combine. Garnish with a few sprigs of parsley. Enjoy with ½ cup of fruit.

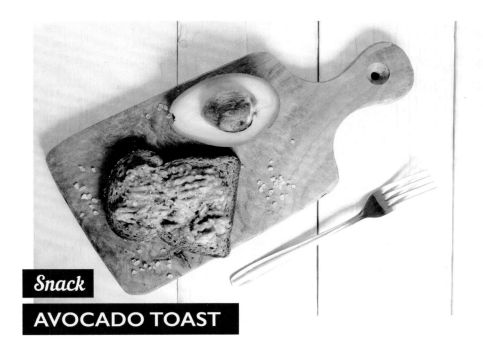

Snack

AVOCADO TOAST

Prep. time 15 minutes | **Cook time** 25 minutes | **1 serving**

INGREDIENTS:

1 slice Ezekiel bread, toasted | 1 tablespoon avocado, mashed |
1 tablespoon hemp seeds | sea salt & black pepper, to taste |
1 tablespoon chia seeds

DIRECTIONS:

Toast Ezekiel bread and top with mashed avocado, hemp seeds, salt & black pepper and chia seeds. Enjoy!

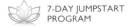

Dinner

BURGER
in a Lettuce Wrap

Prep. time 15 minutes

Cook time 25 minutes

1 serving

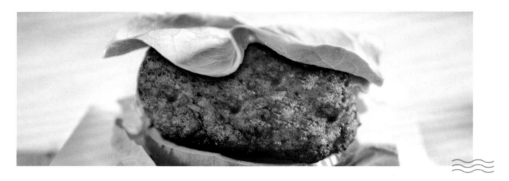

INGREDIENTS:

3 ounces ground grass-fed beef or ground turkey

1-2 leaves of romaine lettuce

½ roma tomato, sliced

¼ red onion, raw

1 tablespoon yellow mustard

½ medium sized sweet potato

1 teaspoon paprika

1 teaspoon sea salt

1 teaspoon black pepper

1 teaspoon garlic or onion powder

1 1/2 tablespoons unrefined coconut oil, melted

DIRECTIONS:

Preheat oven 400°F. Peel sweet potato and cut into thin "french fry" like slices. Cover with ½ tablespoon melted, coconut oil and top with sea salt.

Bake in oven for about 35 minutes or until cooked to desired doneness. While sweet potatoes are cooking, add meat and spices in a large mixing bowl and mix until spices are evenly distributed. Use your hands and form mixture into 1 medium sized patty.

Add remaining coconut oil to pan and cook burger on the stove, over medium heat until cooked through. Place burger on lettuce leaves and top with tomato, onion and mustard. Eat with sweet potato fries on the side.

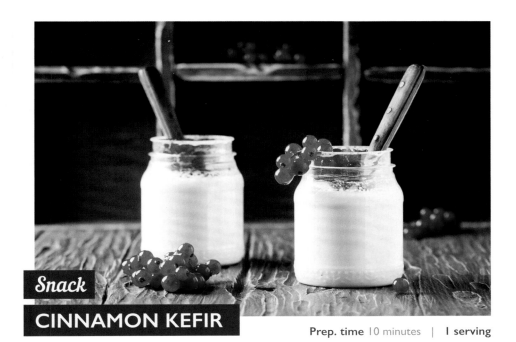

Snack
CINNAMON KEFIR

Prep. time 10 minutes | 1 serving

INGREDIENTS:

3 oz. Plain Kefir | 1 teaspoon Cinnamon | 1 teaspoon Raw Stevia | 1/4 Cup Fresh Raspberries (or fruit of choice)

DIRECTIONS:

Mix all ingredients together in a blender and enjoy.

Men: Creating Your Weekly Menus!

Your success is only 7 days away!

Tips for success when implementing the 7-Day Jumpstart:

- Use ingredients from the list of approved non-inflammatory foods on pages 14-15 to create meals and snacks for your 7 day plan. If you still need a little help, we've created a bonus 7 day PDF with daily meal plans here http://7dayjs.com/program/

- Drink at least 1 gallon of water daily! You can flavor your water with fresh lemon & herbs.

- To jumpstart your metabolism make sure your first meal is within 1 hour of waking up. Eat each meal within 2-3 hours of one another.

- Use the link below to join my 30 day challenge - where I'll share a detailed step by step guide to detox your body, completely done-for-you 30 day meal plans that tells you what to eat and when, highly effective workouts, new meditations, deals, discounts and more.

30 Day Challenge: www.DanetteMay.com/start30dc

Embark on your journey of self-improvement by recording daily events to guide you towards a healthy lifestyle. Record them in a journal or right here. Below are a few ideas to get you started:

What did you eat?

_____
_____
_____

How are you feeling?

_____
_____
_____

What was your workout?

_____

_____

_____

What made you smile today?

_____

_____

_____

Remind yourself of your "why." Write what is in YOUR heart!

_____

_____

_____

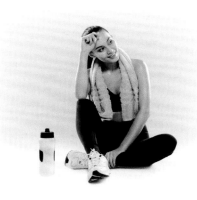

Good things come to those who sweat

Notes

7-DAY JUMPSTART
PROGRAM

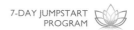

Weekly Menu For Men

Breakfast

- 6 ounces protein
- ½ cup vegetables
- 1 cup carbs
- ½ cup fruit

Snack

- 3 ounces protein
- ½ cup vegetables

Lunch

- 3 ounces protein
- ½ cup vegetables
- ½ cup fruit

Snack

- 3 ounces protein
- ¼ cup carbs
- 1 tablespoon healthy fats

Dinner

- 6 ounces protein
- 1 cup vegetables
- ½ cup carbs
- 1 teaspoon healthy fats

Snack

- 3 ounces protein
- ¼ cup fruit

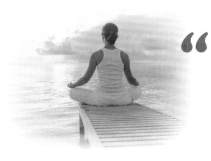

Take care of your body, it's the only place you have to live in

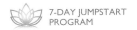

Day One Example Meal Plan For Men

Breakfast

EGGS & SPINACH
with Side of Oatmeal

Prep. time 15 minutes

Cook time 25 minutes

1 serving

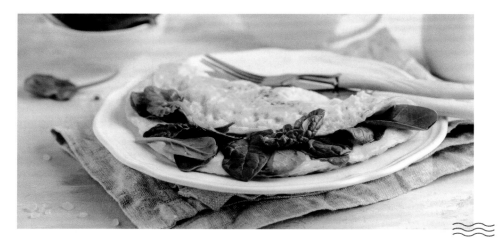

INGREDIENTS:

1/2 cup spinach

1 tablespoon chopped onion

4 eggs

4 sprigs sweet basil

1/2 cup oatmeal

1/2 cup blueberries (or berries of choice)

1-2 teaspoons cinnamon

DIRECTIONS:

Coat skillet with non-stick cooking spray. Place 1/2 cup spinach & 1 tablespoon chopped onion in a skillet over medium heat, cook until wilted. Add 4 eggs, cook until done and top with sweet basil.

Cook 1/2 cup oats according to the package. If you like creamier oatmeal, add water to desired consistency, top with berries and cinnamon.

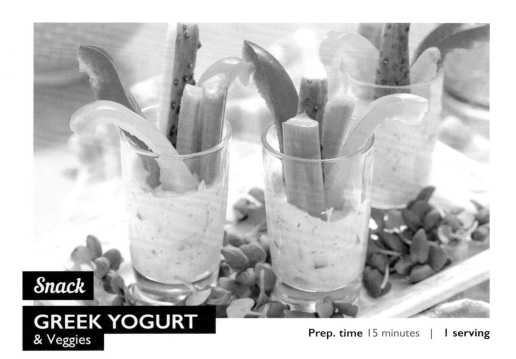

Snack

GREEK YOGURT
& Veggies

Prep. time 15 minutes | **1 serving**

INGREDIENTS:

½ cup plain Greek yogurt | crushed red pepper, to taste | rosemary, to taste | fresh dill, to taste | ½ cup sliced red pepper or vegetable of choice from approved list

DIRECTIONS:

Mix ½ cup plain Greek yogurt with crushed red pepper, rosemary & dill. Enjoy with ½ cup sliced red peppers or other vegetable of choice.

Lunch

GROUND TURKEY
with Warm Fruit Dessert

Prep. time 15 minutes

Cook time 25 minutes

1 serving

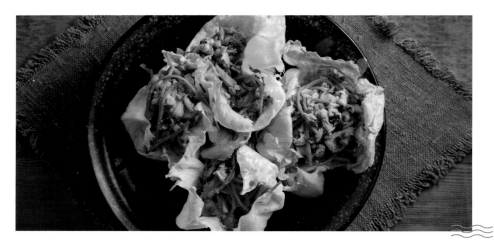

INGREDIENTS:

3 ounces ground turkey

1 teaspoon taco seasoning

½ cup of green lettuce of choice

fresh cilantro, chopped, to taste

½ cup apple or pear

pinch of cinnamon or nutmeg

DIRECTIONS:

Take 3 ounces ground turkey, cook in skillet until fully cooked, add 1 teaspoon taco seasoning. When evenly mixed, scoop turkey meat on ½ cup of greens and top with fresh cilantro.

Slice an apple or a pear, sprinkle with cinnamon or nutmeg. Place in pan and bake for 15 minutes in 350°F. in oven.

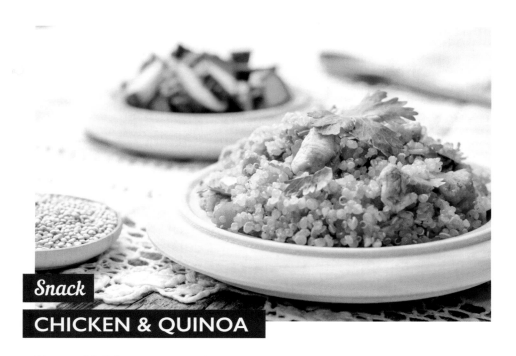

Snack
CHICKEN & QUINOA

Prep. time 15 minutes | **Cook time** 25 minutes | 1 serving

INGREDIENTS:

¼ cup quinoa | 3 ounces cooked chicken, cubed | desired spices and herbs, to taste | 1 tablespoon extra virgin olive oil

DIRECTIONS:

Prepare a batch of quinoa according to packaging. Store in refrigerator and take out ¼ cup and add in 3 ounces cooked chicken breasts, cubed for a snack on the go. When ready to eat, drizzle 1 tablespoon of extra virgin olive oil and fresh spices and herbs.

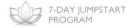

Dinner

SALMON & VEGGIES

Prep. time 15 minutes

Cook time 25 minutes

1 serving

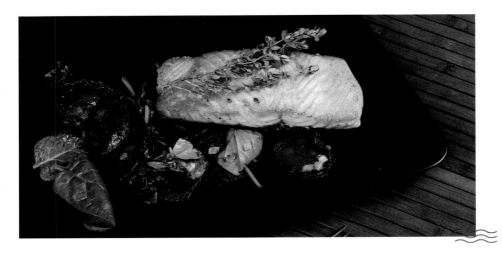

INGREDIENTS:

6 ounces wild caught salmon

1 cup beets or vegetables of choice, steamed

½ cup brown rice

juice from ½ of a lemon

black pepper, to taste

spice of choice (I like curry with this recipe), to taste

1 teaspoon extra virgin olive oil

DIRECTIONS:

Take 6 ounces salmon place in tin foil. Squeeze juice from ½ a lemon on it and top with black pepper. Secure in tin foil and bake at 350 degrees for 30 minutes.

Cook brown rice according to package directions. Add any spice you would like.

Steam 1 cup of beets or vegetables, top with black pepper & 1 teaspoon extra virgin olive oil.

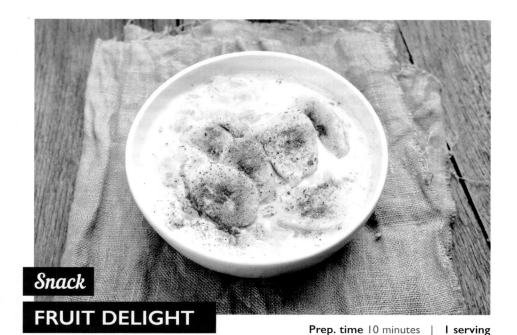

FRUIT DELIGHT

Prep. time 10 minutes | **1 serving**

INGREDIENTS:

½ cup plain Greek yogurt | ¼ cup fruit of choice | cinnamon, to taste | 1 serving of stevia according to package. (choose a natural stevia)

DIRECTIONS:

Mix ½ cup plain Greek yogurt with ¼ cup fruit, sprinkle with cinnamon and stevia. Enjoy!

Notes

Breakfast

TOMATO AVOCADO
& Egg on Toast

Prep. time 15 minutes

Cook time 25 minutes

1 serving

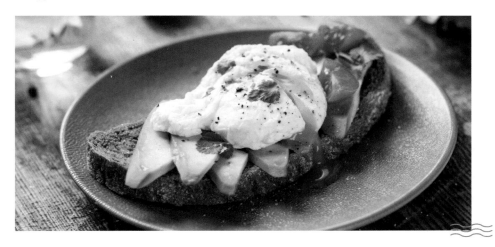

INGREDIENTS:

5 eggs

1/2 avocado

1 roma tomato

2 slices of toasted Ezekiel bread

½ cup fruit of choice

DIRECTIONS:

Coat frying pan with non-stick cooking spray and fry eggs in a pan, over medium heat.

Toast Ezekiel bread, spread avocado on toast. Top with sliced tomato and fried eggs. Serve with ½ cup fruit of choice. Enjoy!

49

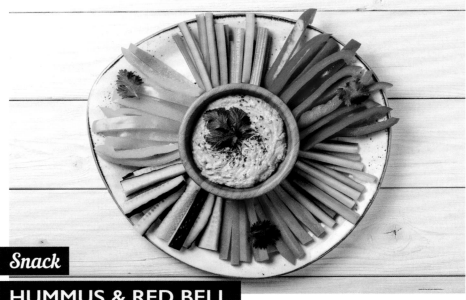

Snack

HUMMUS & RED BELL PEPPER SLICES

Prep. time 15 minutes | **1 serving**

INGREDIENTS:

1/2 cup garbanzo (chickpeas) beans rinsed & drained (reserve 1/8 - 1/4 cup of liquid) | 1 clove garlic | 1 tablespoon tahini | 1 teaspoon freshly squeezed lemon juice | 2 teaspoons extra virgin olive oil | 1/8 - 1/4 teaspoon cumin or chili powder (optional) | 1/4 teaspoon sea salt | pinch of black pepper | 1/2 cup sliced red peppers or vegetable of choice from approved list

DIRECTIONS:

Add garbanzo beans, garlic, tahini, lemon juice, extra virgin olive oil, sea salt, black pepper and 1/8 - 1/4 cup liquid from garbanzo beans. Add more if needed. Blend ingredients together until you get a thick, creamy mixture without any chunks. Eat hummus with 1/2 cup of sliced red pepper or other vegetable of choice. Enjoy!

Lunch

GREEK SALAD

Prep. time 15 minutes

1 serving

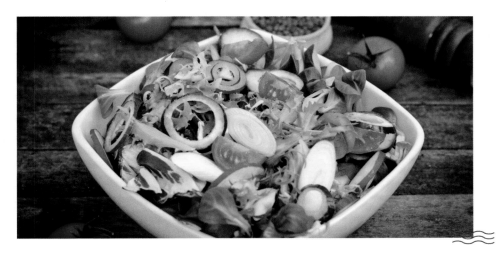

INGREDIENTS:

1 cup romaine lettuce, chopped

8 cherry tomatoes, halved

1/2 cucumber, diced

1 tablespoon red onion, diced

1 tablespoon parsley, chopped

for vegetarians add 2 2/3 cups garbanzo (chickpeas) beans (rinsed & drained)

for meat eaters, add 6 ounces cooked chicken, cubed

DRESSING:

2 tablespoons extra virgin olive oil

2 tablespoons freshly squeezed lemon juice

DIRECTIONS:

Add all salad ingredients into a bowl. In a separate, smaller bowl, mix dressing.

Drizzle dressing over salad and toss to mix.

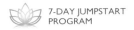

Berries and Nuts

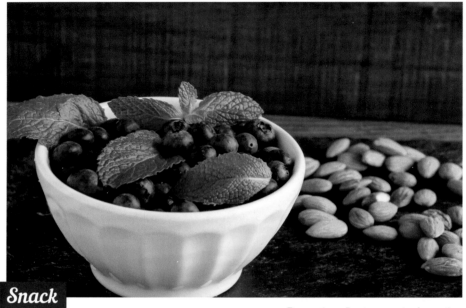

Snack

Prep. time 5 minutes | **I serving**

INGREDIENTS:

¼ cup of raw almonds | ½ cup of berries (blueberries, raspberries or strawberries) | ½ cup Greek yogurt

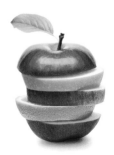

" *Remember when your body is hungry, it wants NUTRIENTS, not calories.* "

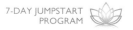

Dinner

CHICKEN
with Broccoli & Rice

Prep. time 15 minutes

Cook time 25 minutes

1 serving

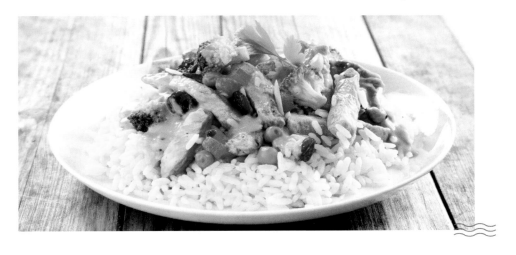

INGREDIENTS:

6 ounces chicken (grilled or cooked in pan)

1 cup broccoli florets

½ cup brown rice or quinoa

1 1/2 cups chicken or vegetable stock

1 teaspoon sea salt

1 teaspoon black pepper

1 tablespoon unrefined coconut oil

juice from ½ of a lemon (optional)

DIRECTIONS:

Cook chicken in a pan with coconut oil until cooked through.

Steam broccoli florets. Cook rice or quinoa according to directions on package using chicken or vegetable stock instead of water to add flavor.

Season meal with sea salt, black pepper and any other preferred spices. Top with lemon juice (optional).

Apples and Peanut Butter

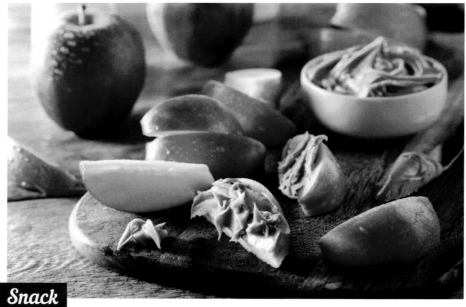

Snack

Prep. time 5 minutes | **I serving**

INGREDIENTS:

½ apple | 2 tablespoons raw peanut or almond butter

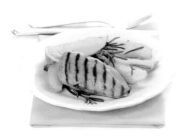

"Every time you eat or drink you are either feeding your body or fighting it"

Notes

Day Three Example For Men

Breakfast

OAT BREAKFAST
with Fruit and Nuts

Prep. time 15 minutes

1 **serving**

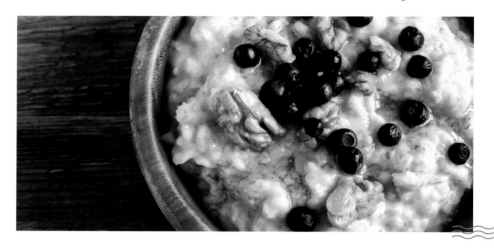

INGREDIENTS:

1 cup old-fashioned oats
(slow cook)

1/2 cup blueberries

¼ cup walnuts

pinch of cinnamon (optional)

1/2 cup vegetables of choice
from approved list

½ cup plain Greek yogurt

DIRECTIONS:

Cook oats according to package.
Top with berries, nuts and pinch of
cinnamon if desired.

Eat with 1/2 cup vegetables and ½ cup
plain greek yogurt.

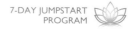

Eggs and Veggies

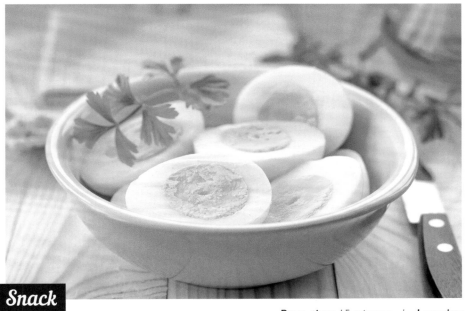

Snack

Prep. time 15 minutes | **1 serving**

INGREDIENTS:

2-3 hard boiled eggs | ½ cup red bell pepper slices

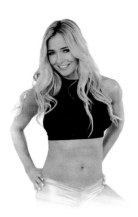

*Eat for the body you want,
not the body you have*

Lunch

QUINOA SALAD

Prep. time 15 minutes

Cook time 25 minutes

1 serving

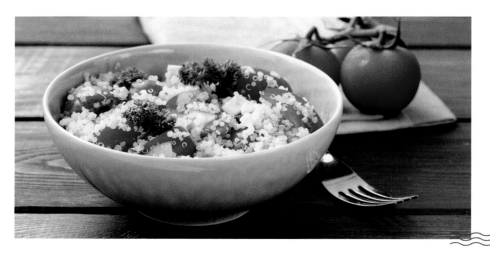

INGREDIENTS:

¼ cup cooked quinoa

¼ cucumber, diced

¼ cup walnuts, raw

¼ red bell pepper, diced

1 tablespoon extra virgin olive oil

2 tablespoons balsamic vinegar

3-4 sprigs of fresh parsley.

sea salt and black pepper, to taste

1/2 cup of fruit from approved list

2 ounces of cooked chicken (cubed)

DIRECTIONS:

Cook quinoa according to directions on the package and allow to cool. Add quinoa, chicken, cucumber, walnuts, and red pepper to a large mixing bowl. Add extra virgin olive oil, balsamic vinegar, salt and black pepper. Toss to combine. Garnish with a few sprigs of parsley.

Enjoy with ½ cup of fruit.

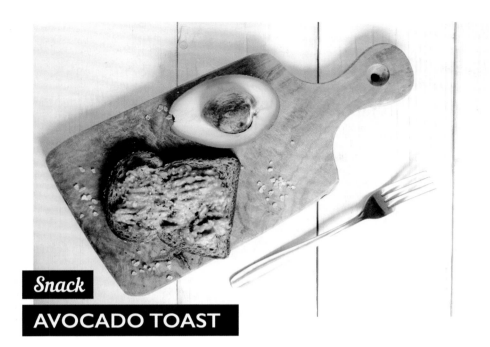

Snack
AVOCADO TOAST

Prep. time 10 minutes | **Cook time** 10 minutes | **1 serving**

INGREDIENTS:

1 slice Ezekiel bread, toasted | 1 tablespoon avocado, mashed |
1 tablespoons hemp seeds | sea salt & black pepper, to taste |
1 tablespoon chia seeds

DIRECTIONS:

Toast Ezekiel bread and top with mashed avocado, hemp seeds, salt & black pepper and chia seeds. Enjoy!

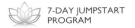

Dinner

BURGER
in a Lettuce Wrap

Prep. time 15 minutes

Cook time 25 minutes

1 serving

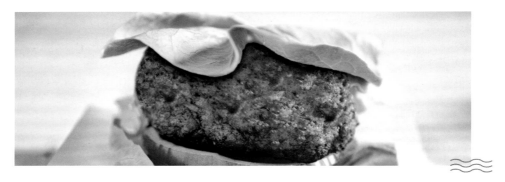

INGREDIENTS:

6 ounces ground grass-fed beef or ground turkey

2-4 leaves of romaine lettuce

1 roma tomato, sliced

½ red onion, raw

1 tablespoon yellow mustard

1 medium sized sweet potato

1 teaspoon paprika

1 teaspoon sea salt

1 teaspoon black pepper

1 teaspoon garlic or onion powder

1 1/2 tablespoons unrefined coconut oil, melted

DIRECTIONS:

Preheat oven 400°F. Peel sweet potato and cut into thin "french fry" like slices. Cover with ½ tablespoon melted, coconut oil and top with sea salt.

Bake in oven for about 35 minutes or until cooked to desired doneness. While sweet potatoes are cooking, add meat and spices in a large mixing bowl and mix until spices are evenly distributed. Use your hands and form mixture into 2 medium sized patties.

Add remaining coconut oil to pan and cook patties on the stove, over medium heat until cooked through. Place burger on lettuce leaves and top with tomato, onion and mustard. Eat with sweet potato fries on the side.

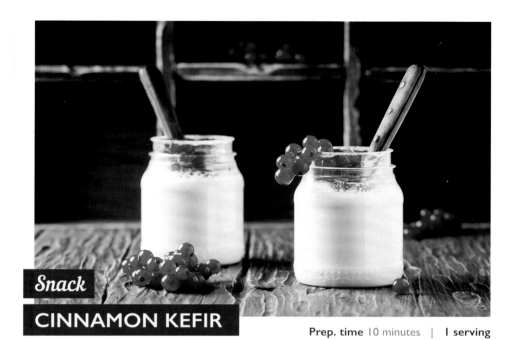

Snack

CINNAMON KEFIR

Prep. time 10 minutes | 1 serving

INGREDIENTS:

3 oz. Plain Kefir | 1 teaspoon Cinnamon | 1 teaspoon Raw Stevia |
1/4 Cup Fresh Raspberries (or fruit of choice)

DIRECTIONS:

Mix all ingredients together in a blender and enjoy.

Notes

7-DAY JUMPSTART
PROGRAM

Why You Need Exercise

As I structure your workouts for the week, I want your body to be able to burn as many calories as it can efficiently, without having you work out 2 or more hours a day. Actually, through recent research, we learned that working out less can often result in more! Spending 20-30 minutes working out using this program can burn more calories than if you were to use the treadmill or go on a run for over an hour. I know that is music to your ears, so I have constructed the most efficient, fat decreasing, lean muscle gaining workouts you can get in 7 days by incorporating HIIT training and strength training.

What Is HIIT?

HIIT (high-intensity interval training) is cardio performed at such an intense level that your body will spend the rest of the day expending energy to recover from the ass-kicking you gave it. Commonly referred to as EPOC (excess post-exercise oxygen consumption), and it means that you consume a great deal more oxygen recovering from the exercises than you would have if you'd just done a steady-state workout (steady-state meaning hours of cardio on machines). You will be burning up to nine times more fat while sitting on the couch later in the evening than you would have if you'd spent an hour on the treadmill at a moderate pace. I am talking about intense training. You will need to push yourself out of the comfort zone you have gotten used to and challenge yourself. If you are willing to do this, I can guarantee that you will spend less than half the time you usually do on those machines and get much leaner in the process.

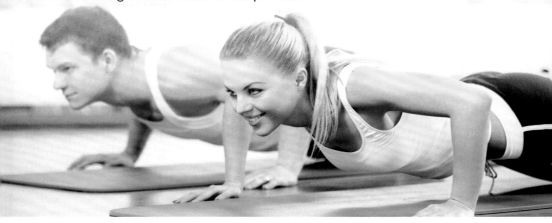

Benefits of HIIT

HIIT training has many benefits, in addition to the reduction in training time. First, this type of training is far superior to steady-state exercises when it comes to increasing your VO2 max, which is the maximum amount of oxygen you can uptake during exercise; meaning that you'll be in much better shape.Next, when you perform long-duration, moderate-intensity exercise, you can put yourself in a catabolic state in where you will start losing muscle mass. That's right! Some of that hard-earned muscle will begin tearing itself down in your quest to get lean.

Strength Training Benefits

Strength training will add definition to your muscles and give both men and women a more toned, fit, lean body. Before I expand on the benefits, I would like to debunk a myth right now that a lot of women have. You will not bulk up with strength training. Eating foods outlined in the 7-Day Jumpstart and by following the workouts, your waist will get smaller, and your thighs will slim down. Men, on the other hand, will get bigger in all the right places. It has a lot to do with the hormone, testosterone.

Men have naturally higher amounts than women. The more muscle your body has, the higher your metabolism is going to be. It takes a whole lot more energy to carry and sustain muscle than it does fat, hence you will transform your physique into a fit body type. Working out with weights does so much more!

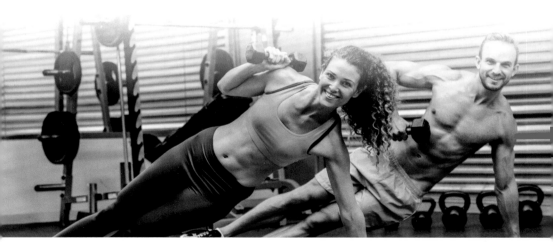

1. **Strength training protects bone health and muscle mass.**

   After puberty, whether you are a man or a woman, you begin to lose about 1 percent of your bone and muscle strength every year. "One of the best ways to stop, prevent, and even reverse bone and muscle loss is to add strength training to your workouts," advises Troy Tuttle, MS, an exercise physiologist at the University of Texas Medical School in Houston.

2. **Strength training makes you stronger and fitter.**

   Strength training is also called resistance training because it involves strengthening and toning your muscles by contracting them against a resisting force. There are two types of resistance training: Isometric resistance involves contracting your muscles against a non-moving object, such as against the floor in a push-up.

   Isotonic strength training involves contracting your muscles through a range of motion as in weightlifting. Both make you stronger and can get you into better shape. Remember that with strength training your muscles will need time to recover, so alternate days. Always take some time to warm up and cool down after strength training.

3. **Strength training helps you develop better body mechanics.**

   Strength training has benefits that go well beyond the appearance of toned muscles. Your balance and coordination will improve, as well as your posture. More importantly, if you have poor flexibility and balance, strength training can reduce your risk of falling by as much as 40 percent, a crucial benefit, especially as you get older.

4. **Strength training plays a role in disease prevention.**

   Studies have documented the many wellness benefits of strength training. If you have arthritis, strength training can be as effective as medication in decreasing arthritis pain. Strength training can help post-menopausal women increase their bone density and reduce the risk of bone fractures. And for the over 14 million Americans with type 2 diabetes, strength training along with other healthy lifestyle changes can help improve glucose control!

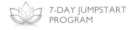

5. **Strength training boosts energy levels and improves your mood.**

   Strength training will elevate your level of endorphins (natural opiates produced by the brain), which will make you feel great. As if that isn't enough to convince you, strength training has also been shown to be a great antidepressant, to help you sleep better, and to improve your overall quality of life.

6. **Strength training translates to more calories burned.**

   You burn calories during strength training, and your body continues to burn calories AFTER strength training, in a process called "physiologic homework." More calories are used to make and maintain muscle than fat, and in fact, strength training can boost your metabolism by 15 percent; that can jumpstart a weight loss plan.

Getting Started With Strength Training

Please don't limit yourself to thinking that lifting weights, using expensive machines, or a gym membership is the only way to do strength training.

Push-ups, jump squats, lunges, and mountain climbers are all examples of exercises that provide strength training. Who doesn't want to look better, feel better, and live a longer, healthier life?

The 7-Day Jumpstart is going to get you started!

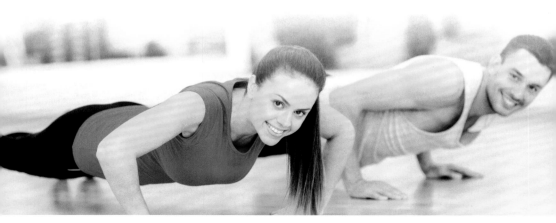

Warm Up

5-10 minutes of movement until your body gets warm or sweat starts to form. Do not skip this phase. You will reduce the risk of injury, which can happen with body blast workouts. Your muscles need to be warm, engaged, and ready to pick up the tempo during the blast phase.

Some examples of warm-up options are jumping jacks, jogging in place, punch and jabs, dancing, jump rope or using a stationary elliptical or bike. If you prefer to follow along with us, you can access warm-ups via video here: www.7dayjs.com/program

Cool Down

5-10 minutes of movement bringing your heart rate down and back to a comfortable talking state. You can walk, lightly jog in place or bring your knees up and down while gently swinging your arms.

To watch all of our workouts on video,
www.7dayjs.com/program

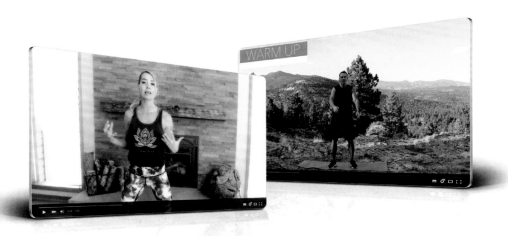

Body Fat Blast Workout

Plank on the Floor

(or plank on the ball with alternating leg lift).

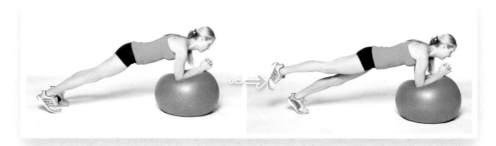

How To: Place shoulders in direct line with elbows. Keep glutes in line with your spine. You can lift and lower each leg one at a time for added balance and strength.

Goal: a total of 30 seconds

One Leg Scissor

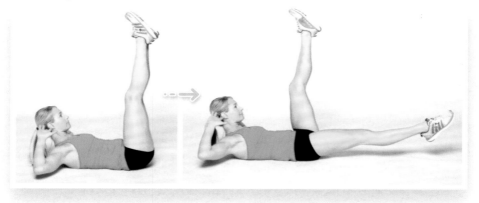

How To: Pull abs in towards your spine. Keep legs straight. Begin by alternating legs. Lower legs just low enough before you lower back lifts off the floor. Keep belly button pulled in toward your spine throughout the movement.

Goal: a total of 20 leg scissors

Jump Squat

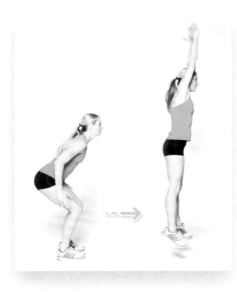

How To: Make sure to land softly through the heel of your feet. Explode up in the air, land softly, sticking glutes back and down.

Land on your feet while resting on your heels before you explode again. Modification: if you have bad knees or are a beginner you can do the squat without the jump.

Goal: a total of 20 reps

Tricep Push Up With Rotation

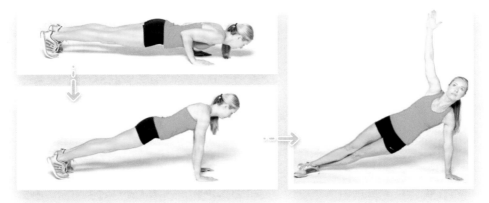

How To: Begin in a push-up position with your body in alignment from head to heels. Keep shoulders in line with your wrists. Lower your body, then raise back up slowly. Lift one arm into the sky while rotating your body to an open position. Repeat on the other side. Modification: you can drop to your knees.

Goal: a total of 12 tricep push-ups

Power Frog Jumps

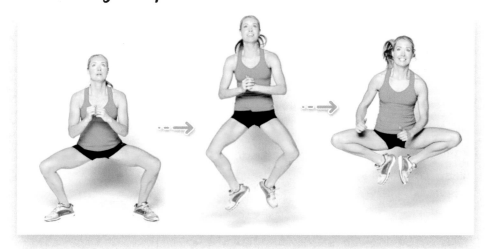

How To: Explode in the air and touch heels together. Land softly with feet wide and toes pointed slightly out. Modification: don't jump, but keep legs wide, toes turned out then lift and lower through your heels.

Goal: 20 total. *You will repeat this sequence 3 times.*

Crab Touch

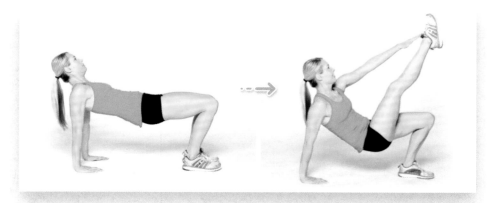

How To: Keep your glutes up and body in alignment. Reach arm up to opposite foot. Touch the top of your toe.

Goal: a total of 10 on each side

HIIT Workout

- I minute walk
- I minute sprint
- Repeat this sequence until you reach 20 minutes

The key is to recover enough to push during the I minute push phase.

Modification: if you cannot sprint due to bad knees, you can do this workout biking or swimming. Your push phase, if you are biking or swimming, will be 2 minutes instead of I minute.

Weekly Workout

Workout Videos: www.7dayjs.com/program

DAY 1	DAY 2	DAY 3	DAY 4
Prep day: Getting Started	Warm-Up Body Fat Blast Workout Cool Down	HIIT Workout	Warm-Up Body Fat Blast Workout Cool Down

DAY 5	DAY 6	DAY 7	DAY 8
Rest Day	HIIT Workout	Warm-Up Body Fat Blast Workout Cool Down	HIIT Workout

Selecting Quality Sourced Animal Protein

Animal protein can sometimes get a bad reputation, especially with an increasing awareness of the treatment of animals, growth hormones injected and the health of the animals in factory farming. Also, we have seen the trends toward the organic plant-based and vegetarian or vegan foods increasing in the past few years. I promote a very balanced diet that is of a high proportion of plant-based foods, but I also include clean, quality sourced animal products.

I want to provide a bit of education around how to source high-quality animal products so that you know how to make healthier decisions when it comes to meat and dairy selections.

Beef or Steak

Cows are meant to eat grass. Cows in America are typically fed grains, injected with growth hormones to fatten and bulk them up to produce more meat and taste better. Cows should be allowed to roam in grassy pastures. However, in factory farming, cows are stuck in small compounds and sometimes cages next to each other, making it easy for bacteria and viruses to spread. To prevent the spreading of disease among the cows, they are provided antibiotics. When you consume the cow, you are eating the hormones, the antibiotics and whatever other toxins in their bodies.

Solution: BUY ORGANIC AND GRASS-FED MEAT WHENEVER AVAILABLE. If you cannot afford it or it is not available, then think about reducing your intake of meat. I recommend researching local grass-fed farms in your area and consider buying meat from them! Another option is to purchase your meat online from companies like Butcher Box at www.ButcherBoxDiscounts.com - who deliver grass-fed meats and organic poultry right to your doorstep!

Chicken

Chickens are meant to roam free through grassy pastures. Factory farmed chickens are put in tiny cages, not able to move. They also contract diseases and are injected with antibiotics, as well as growth hormones to plump them up. These chickens then lay eggs. We eat the chicken and their eggs.

Solution: BUY ORGANIC PASTURE raised or free-range chicken whenever possible.

Eggs

The best quality eggs are pasture-raised; where chickens are free to roam and forage in open pastures like they are supposed to. My favorite brand is Vital Farms Pasture-Raised eggs that you can find at many grocery stores today. A local farmer who sells pasture-raised eggs is an excellent choice, too! You will notice the egg yolk is much more vibrant in color and full of nutrients!

Fish

Fish are meant to swim freely in the ocean and not be farmed in close quarters with thousands of other fish. Farmed fish not only lose a lot of the beneficial nutrients, but they can also spread disease in these tight quarters.

Solution: BUY WILD CAUGHT salmon and fish WHENEVER POSSIBLE. Wild caught salmon is MUCH richer in color compared to farmed salmon, which have food dyes added making the salmon more colorful.

The overall summary is, choose food choices as close to nature as possible. Avoid packaged and processed food when given a choice. If your meat comes from animals that are raised as they would be in nature, then they're safe to eat. I recommend looking up local farms in your area and source your meat from there.

Knowing where your food comes from is essential, and when eating out, it's difficult to know. I encourage my clients to cook at home as much as possible so that you have better control over the quality of what you consume. Remove foods you crave from your home. If it's not visible, you are less likely to be tempted!

Double-check to make sure your goals are measurable and realistic. Don't try to overhaul everything all at once. Focus on a few small, but mighty changes. The 7-Day Jumpstart has done this for you. We have provided all the tools you need to be successful. All you need to do is focus on eating foods from the list provided and follow the workouts and give it your best. Then you can sit back and watch the beginning of your body and mind transformations.

Enlist the help of meaningful people in your life for support. Tell others about your goal and see if they would like to join you. Especially, tell those living with you. Ask them to support you and to help you in this quest for optimal health.

We also recommend that you educate yourself! Take the time to read through all of the content in this book so that you understand WHY this program works and how to make healthier choices. We also provide additional tips and tools that you can implement in your life that will support you on your journey to a healthier and happier you!

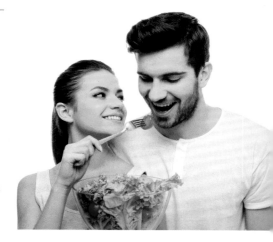

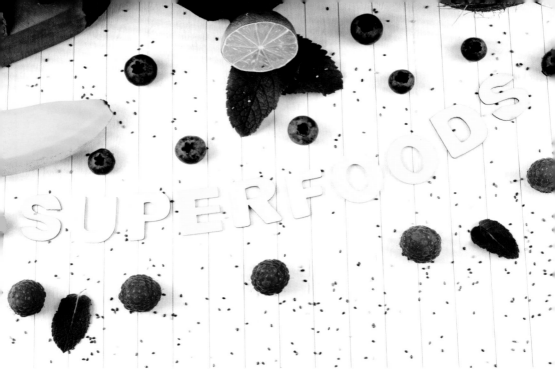

Introducing the Superfoods

Superfoods are nutrient-dense foods that can deliver specific health benefits. Many of these foods lower and regulate blood sugar levels which is an important factor to slow down the development of body fat, the aging process, and wrinkles.

Including superfoods in your diet may offer the following benefits:

- Prevents or reduces inflammation
- Burns body fat
- Decreases cholesterol

- Decreases blood pressure
- Promotes digestive health
- Regulates blood sugar

Acai Berry

Packed with antioxidants, amino acids, and essential fatty acids! Acai berries are rich with fiber, which slows your absorption of carbohydrates. It controls blood sugar levels to help control insulin spikes *(which in the end decreases fat gain)* As a bonus; all the antioxidants help with premature aging! Win!

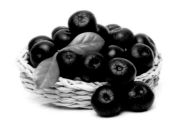

Buckwheat

High in protein, amino acids, and essential minerals. Buckwheat decreases high blood pressure and LDL cholesterol. Reducing LDL (lousy) cholesterol decreases body fat!

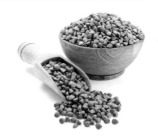

Beans and Lentils

High in fiber, and folic acid. These little guys help with anti-aging and decreasing body fat! Fiber helps with carbohydrate absorption, as well as satiation and controls your blood sugar levels which keep insulin spikes down.

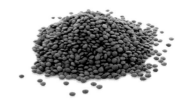

Nuts and Seeds

Raw & unsalted nuts/seeds decreases risk of heart disease, high in omega-3 and omega-6 and also in vitamin E. This healthy fat helps regulate fat burning hormones. Nuts and seeds will help control appetite and cravings, too!

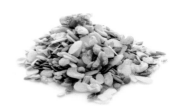

Chia Seeds

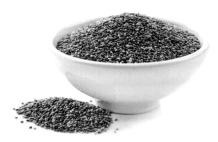

High in fiber, omega-3 fatty acids, calcium, magnesium, phosphorous and protein. The gelatinous coating chia develops when exposed to liquid can help prevent blood sugar spikes and support with blood sugar regulation. Chia seeds are great for heart health by lowering blood pressure and cholesterol. They are also one of the few plant-based sources of a complete protein.

Ways to include them in your diet: add to your morning smoothie, make chia pudding by mixing with unsweetened almond or unsweetened coconut milk, soak in water or tea and drink, sprinkle on a salad, add to baking recipes.

Hemp Seeds

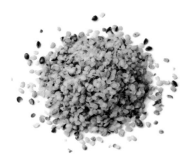

Have a balanced omega-6 to omega-3 fatty acids ratio. They have 3 grams of protein per serving. Contain vitamins A, E, D and many B vitamins. They are good for heart health and lowering blood pressure, and control blood sugar levels. Hemp seeds are a great addition to add to your morning smoothie, sprinkle over oatmeal or on top of a salad.

Plain Greek Yogurt and Plain Kefir

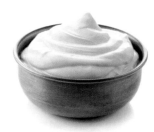

These low inflammatory foods help with stomach bulge by decreasing inflammation in your abdominals! Both contain naturally occurring probiotics due to the fermentation process which supports gut health. And fight against infectious diseases and increases immune function. POW!

Allium Group

Onions, scallions, shallots - This group of foods will not only flavor your meals and satisfy your senses, but they will also give you an extra boost of nutrients! Foods from the allium family are known to support cardiovascular health, reducing cholesterol levels, lowering blood pressure, and they are also known to have anti-inflammatory effects on the body!

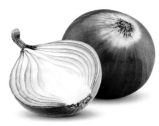

Wheatgrass

Wheatgrass is an amazingly potent little plant! It has an impressive amount of minerals, as well as the entire array of B-vitamins, vitamin A, vitamin C, E and K. The juice of wheatgrass contains up to 70% chlorophyll, which is a helpful blood builder. Chlorophyll also has antioxidants and acts as a free radical scavenger. It cleanses our bodies, reduces inflammation, supports eliminating toxins and helps with the reduction of excess belly and thigh fat.

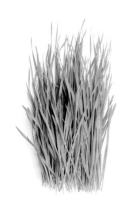

Water

Water is a superfood due to its healing powers and daily importance to our overall health. Our body is made up of 70% water! Toxins hide in fat cells and water is a flushing agent. Water is also responsible for lubricating our organs.

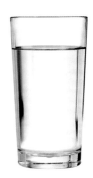

Benefits of Low Inflammatory Foods

Benefits	How It Helps You
Increases production of collagen and elastin	Genuine deep, lasting youthful beauty
Repairs scars, injuries, and wrinkles	Younger healthier looking, fast healing, restores total health
Increases circulation	Clarity of mind, energy flow, heart health, longevity, better sex
Experience rapid wound repair	Quicker recovery, fast track back to perfect health
Develops a radiant, supple appearance to skin that you haven't seen since your youth	Healthy glow, confidence, attractiveness, beauty
Decreases inflammation in every organ system	Reduced arthritis pain, decreased swollen abdomen
Increases efficiency of metabolism, resulting in cellular repair	Improved weight loss & muscle growth, burn fat, build lean muscle mass, look better
Elevates mood	Whatever level you are at right now, you will feel even better. Which means better performance & better success

Why Anti-Inflammatory Foods are Used in the 7-Day Jumpstart

It seems we're all trying to find that "magic pill" that delays the natural aging process and burns stubborn belly fat. Put an anti-aging or fat burning label on most any product, and it flies off the shelves.

If you're trying to look your best without going under the knife; the secret is closer than you think. It's a place you most likely visit weekly. The grocery store! Walk down the aisles, and you will see healing fruits, vegetables, spices, green tea, and a host of other healthful foods that are rich in antioxidants, fat burning components, and anti-inflammatory compounds.

Weight Gain and Inflammatory Foods

Science has sufficiently proven that fat cells do cause inflammation, but it appears there is also a possibility that inflammation itself triggers weight gain. Inflammation has been shown to affect a specific part of the brain (the hypothalamus), causing it to become insulin and leptin resistant.

Whether fat causes inflammation or inflammation causes fat, the critical factor that needs to be understood in any weight loss program is; decrease inflammation and increase cells' sensitivity to insulin and leptin.

To do this one must eliminate foods that are inflammatory, such as sugar and hydrogenated oils, as well as foods that cause an allergic reaction. The focus must be on a diet filled with organic fruits, vegetables, spices and whole grains, which are all naturally anti-inflammatory.

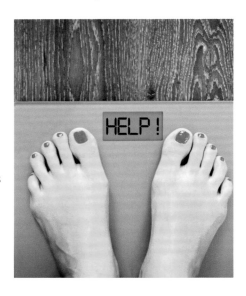

Focusing on processed "low-fat" and "diet" foods may lower the calorie count, but these foods are typically pro-inflammatory, which explains why they don't help with weight loss. They also aren't satiating, and some of the chemicals in these foods trigger hunger signals, making you eat more.

Unlocking the secret to releasing stubborn belly fat indeed lies in the foods you eat, not just exercising and eating less.

Aging and Inflammatory Foods

The signs of aging include not only wrinkles, but also memory loss, decreased brain function, and an increased risk for chronic diseases such as heart disease, osteoporosis, and cancer. Healthy aging is known as living a longer, healthier life. Many studies have documented the link between a healthy diet and prevention of age-related or chronic diseases. Adopting a healthy lifestyle that includes regular physical activity, adequate rest, avoiding tobacco, and a diet full of clean, healthy foods and beverages can be the best defense against aging. "Dietary choices are critical to delay the onset of aging and age-related diseases, and the sooner you start, the greater the benefit," says Susan Moores, RD, a spokesman for the American Dietetic Association.

Antioxidants and Inflammation

All foods fit into three categories: pro-inflammatory, neutral, or anti-inflammatory. You can reverse fat storage and slow aging at the cellular level by choosing foods that are anti-inflammatory and rich in antioxidants.

Body changes may be reversed by consuming foods and beverages that are rich in a variety of compounds, including antioxidants, and foods that are anti-inflammatory, such as cold-water fish and richly colored fruits and vegetables.

On the other hand, foods classified as pro-inflammatory can accelerate weight gain and aging.

If we eat large amounts of hydrogenated oils or trans fatty acids, sugars, and starches, insulin levels surge and trigger an anti-inflammatory response and accelerate the aging process and fat production.

Making smart lifestyle choices are within your reach and are among the best things you can do to lose weight, help prevent disease and slow the aging process.

Therefore, it is important we eat foods that are protective against inflammation. Our ancestors ate a varied diet of plant and animal foods based on local environment and availability. It makes sense we should, too! Here is a breakdown of components we should include in our diet every day.

Foods rich in omega-3 fatty acids

Animal Sources: wild salmon, anchovies, mackerel & sardines
Plant Sources: hemp, chia seeds, flaxseed meal and walnuts

Research shows that omega-3 fatty acids reduce inflammation and may help lower the risk of chronic diseases such as heart disease, cancer, and arthritis. Omega-3 fatty acids are highly concentrated in the brain and appear to be essential for cognitive *(brain memory and performance)* and behavioral function. In fact, infants who do not get enough omega-3 fatty acids from their mothers during pregnancy are at risk for developing vision and nerve problems. Symptoms of omega-3 fatty acid deficiency include fatigue, poor memory, dry skin, heart problems, mood swings or depression, and poor circulation.

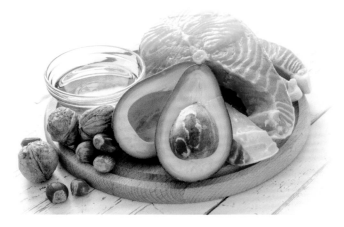

Colorful antioxidant rich vegetables

Choose dark leafy greens like spinach and kale; broccoli and cauliflower; sea vegetables like kelp; red peppers, sweet potatoes, and cabbage.

These vegetables contain anti-inflammatory, anti-cancer phytonutrients that help detoxify the body, which translates into a better functioning metabolism and reduce free radical damage.

Monounsaturated fats

Plants sources include avocado, raw soaked nuts (almonds, cashews, pecans, macadamia) and olive oils. Eating monounsaturated fats reduces inflammation by interfering with leukotrienes (naturally produced molecules that contribute to inflammation).

Spices

Which include turmeric, curry, ginger, garlic and chili peppers. These spices inhibit pro-inflammatory compounds. Turmeric contains curcumin which inhibits enzymes that participate in the synthesis of inflammatory substances in the body.

The natural anti-inflammatory activity of curcumin is comparable in strength to steroidal drugs, and some non-steroidal medicines but does not have the same dangerous side effects. Chili peppers contain the phytochemical capsaicin which reduces levels of substance P, the compound in the body that triggers inflammation and pain impulses from the central nervous system.

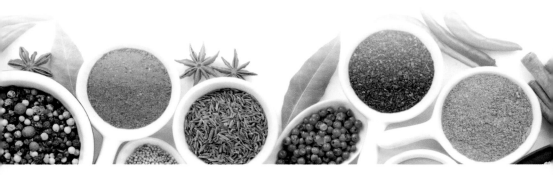

Why Water is Important for Fat Loss

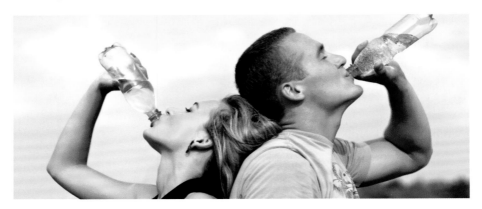

It is time to educate you about the many benefits of water as we tend to forget how important water consumption is to reaching our goals. Our goal is to consume ¾ to a gallon of water each day! Water will aid in weight loss by flushing fat from your body!

Did you know that not drinking enough plain water can be as harmful to your heart as smoking? The benefits from drinking plain water reportedly surpass moderate drinking of wine, taking aspirin and other preventive measures.

Drinking 5 glasses of water daily can decrease the risk of colon cancer by up to 45%, can slash the risk of breast cancer by up to 79%, and can reduce the risk of bladder cancer by up to 50%! Amazing, right?

Preliminary research indicates that consuming 8-10 glasses of water daily could significantly ease back pain and joint pain for up to 80% of sufferers. Lack of water is the number one trigger for daytime fatigue.

A mere 2% drop in body water can cause fuzzy short-term memory, trouble with basic math, and difficulty focusing on the computer screen. In 37% of Americans, the body's thirst mechanism is so weak that it is often mistaken for hunger. One glass of water can shut down midnight hunger pangs for almost 100% of dieters tested in a University of Washington study.

And last, but certainly not least, mild dehydration will slow down one's metabolism as much as 3%.

Inflammation and Gut Health

There is much more information coming out these days about the connection of our gut with our brain and immune system.

Many people do not know that:
75-80% of our immune system is in our gut!
AND
85-90% of our serotonin and serotonin receptors are in our gut, too!

So this means that an unhealthy gut can lead to:

- Low immune function (getting sick easily)

- Mood Swings

- Increase in autoimmune symptoms

- Depression

- Brain fog

- Increased susceptibility to disease

An unhealthy gut can be related to autism and other mental illnesses.

What causes an Unhealthy Gut?

Yep, you guessed it: inflammation in the body! We cause inflammation in our gut from eating inflammatory foods, food sensitivities, stress and gut infections such as bacterial overgrowth, yeast, and parasites. When we experience inflammation in our gut, it interferes with our digestion and absorption of nutrients and can cause unwanted weight gain.

The good thing is we have the power to make healthier choices that can support our gut health and immune system.

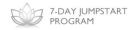

And this is why during the 7-Day Jumpstart, we are focusing on eating non-inflammatory foods! The purpose is to reduce inflammation, by consuming foods that are easily digestible so that we can absorb all of the beneficial nutrients we are eating!

Below are a few steps to support gut health:

1. Reduce inflammatory foods in your diet like food additives in processed & packaged foods, sugar, processed vegetable oils, refined flours, artificial sweeteners, excess consumption of alcohol and trans fats.

2. Include anti-inflammatory food in your diet like leafy green vegetables, ginger, turmeric, broccoli, blueberries, raw walnuts, salmon (most of the foods in our meals for the seven days!)

3. Include fermented foods in your diet like kefir which is full of naturally occurring probiotics, and nutrients that help balance your healthy gut flora and boost the immune system.

When we reduce the inflammation in our body, our body systems perform at more optimal levels which, can support in weight loss, better digestion, better mood and an enhanced immune system so that we can fight off infection!

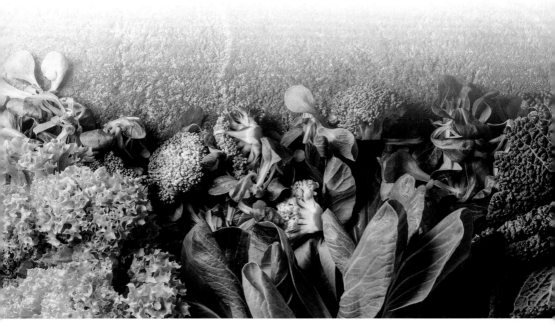

Stress and Inflammation

One of the causes of inflammation in our body is STRESS! Chances are, if you are human, you experience SOME level of stress regularly – and for some of you, likely on a daily basis. It is important to understand the effect of stress on the body.

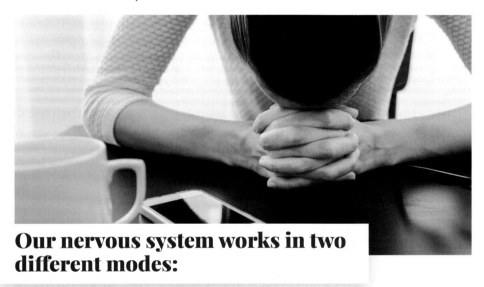

Our nervous system works in two different modes:

1. Parasympathetic (rest and digest) and
2. Sympathetic (fight or flight).

The parasympathetic nervous system is responsible for maintaining homeostasis (balance) in the body. It keeps our body temperature at normal levels, keeps our heart rate down, our blood pressure down. The sympathetic nervous system controls the body's response to a perceived "threat," throwing our body into "fight or flight mode" - preparing our body to stay and fight or run away from the perceived threat.

Back during the Paleolithic era, our bodies were put in fight or flight mode when clear and present danger arose – for example, being chased by a tiger or bear in the forest or perhaps if someone was trying to harm you.

Unfortunately, in our modern day, our sympathetic nervous system is activated almost on a daily basis - someone cuts you off on the freeway, you argue with someone, you have a stressful deadline, a stressful job, an important meeting, or you are running late. Even watching violent movies can turn on our sympathetic nervous system.

So what happens when our body goes into the sympathetic mode? Adrenaline is released, our adrenals start pumping cortisol, our heart rate increases, blood pressure rises, we become short of breath. Our muscles constrict and tighten, our digestive system shuts down, our neurotransmitters and sex hormones go all over the map, and our bodies create inflammation to protect us. Some people get headaches, body aches or pain, diarrhea, acne, anxiety, ulcers, hernias, inflammation, bloating, heart palpitations, etc. It's easy to see that the consistent push into fight or flight mode can have a detrimental effect on our bodies over time - even leading to things like heart disease and cancer due to the repeated physiological stress.

Tips to Reduce Stress in Your Life

Sleep

IMPORTANCE OF SLEEP FOR A HEALTHY LIFESTYLE:

Sleep is important and often overlooked in most weight loss programs. Our bodies need adequate sleep to rest and digest. Most individuals typically need between 7-9 hours of sleep to feel fully rested. According to the Centers for Disease Control and Prevention, more than 35 percent of people are sleep deprived. Sleep deprivation has been shown to not only increase inflammation in the body but also get in the way of losing weight.

Lack of Sleep and Weight Loss

Our bodies produce two hormones that regulate hunger in the body: leptin and ghrelin. Leptin is created in your fat cells and sends signals to your brain that you have enough fat and can eat less or not eat at all, which in turn decreases hunger. Ghrelin is produced in the stomach lining and typically increases hunger and appetite. Both leptin and ghrelin are needed to lose weight, and it's important to maintain a healthy balance. When we do not get adequate amounts of sleep, this creates an imbalance and which can cause us to produce less leptin, and more ghrelin. We then wake up feeling hungry and less satiated throughout the day and end up eating more than we need to, leading to weight gain.

When we provide our body with a good night of sleep, we experience a multitude of health benefits including:

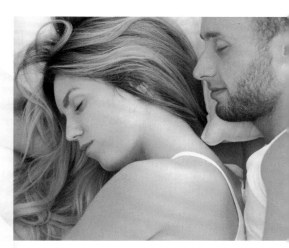

- Lower inflammation

- Support in weight loss

- More energy

- More motivation in life

- Motivation to work out

The stress reducing tips below will help with overall sleep quality. Also, we recommend the following:

- Reduce coffee to 1 cup per day, in the morning. Avoid coffee after 3 pm as coffee has an 8 hour half life – meaning that 8 hours after consumption there is still 50% of it in your system which can affect sleep.

- Drink herbals teas before bed that supports in calming the body. We recommend chamomile, lavender, valerian root or lemon balm.

- Reduce alcohol consumption – especially high sugary alcohols like wine in the evening.

- Avoid sweet snacks or sugary desserts after dinner.

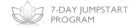

Workout

Working out is such an incredible way to combat the daily stress of life. When we are stressed, our bodies contract and tighten and the best way to release the stiffness in our bodies is to MOVE! When we move our bodies, we support them in lubricating our joints and increasing our range of motion. Working out also provides us with a mental, physical and emotional release!

Below are additional ways working out can support stress reduction:

Increases endorphins – physical activity increases production of endorphins which are our brain's "feel good" neurotransmitters. Have you ever noticed you feel good after a workout? This is the body's natural high we experience after movement!

Moving meditation – a workout can be used as a moving meditation. While you are moving your body, you are bringing all your awareness to your workout or your movement. It brings you to the present moment and calms the mind. When we are focused on our workout, we are not often thinking about our day to day stress.

Enhances mood – because we release endorphins when we work out and "feel" good after, this also enhances our mood. We can approach the day in a happy state and can more easily navigate conflict, thereby reducing stress.

Sleep support – people who work out, typically experience better sleep. By using up energy stored during the day, it helps your bodies natural cortisol rhythm so that it comes down at night and you experience restful sleep.

I have included multiple workouts in the 7-Day Jumpstart because I know how important working out is to supplement any nutrition program. If you get the nutrition, without the movement, you will not see the same results. And working out is also such an incredible way to reduce stress, and consequently, inflammation!

Yoga & Meditations

Practice Yoga

Yoga has been shown to provide a variety of benefits, including stress reduction. The practice of yoga brings you to the present moment by connecting your body, and your mind. By focusing on the flow of your body and the pace of your breathing, the mind follows, quieting the noise and the chatter we typically experience from day to day. Yoga and other mindfulness techniques such as deep breathing and meditation have also been shown to suppress or reverse the production of pro-inflammatory gene expression which can reduce inflammation and reduce the risk of developing diseases linked to inflammation.

Yoga poses are specific and very therapeutic for the physical and energetic bodies. Typically poses that reduce stress are also the same poses we want to focus on to support our sleep. These poses balance and calm the nervous system and bring the body back into homeostasis; when you adopt a regular yoga practice, whether at home or in a studio, you can cultivate peace of the body and the mind.

Below are some simple yoga poses to reduce stress and help you sleep. You can even do them from your bed!

Child's Pose

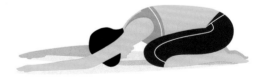

Begin on all fours. Bring the soles of your feet together, and your knees apart. Shift your weight back to your heels, and walk your arms out straight in front of you. Forehead comes down to your mat or your bed. Relax in Child's Pose for up to 3 minutes.

Butterfly

In a seated position, bring the soles of the feet together, making a diamond shape with your legs. Legs can be pulled in close toward the body or for more comfort bring them further out, making the diamond larger. Take a deep breath and slowly come forward with a flat back. You can pause here, or you have the option to round the spine, letting the head hang down toward the feet.

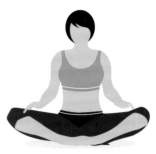

Reclined Bound Angle

Lay down on your back. Option to place a pillow behind your head. Bring the soles of your feet together and allow your knees to fall to the sides, making a diamond shape with your legs. Hold up to 3 minutes or until you start to feel discomfort.

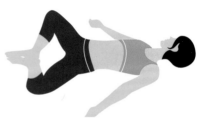

Spinal Twist

Lie down on your back. Bend both knees; feet are planted on your mat or your bed. Allow both knees to fall to the right-hand side. Left-arm reaches straight out behind you, and your gaze follows the extended arm. Hold up to 3 minutes and then switch sides. Bringing the knees back to center and into the chest. Shift the weight from side to side, massaging out the lower back and then allow the knees to drop to the left-hand side. Right arm stretches out behind you, and your gaze follows the extended arm.

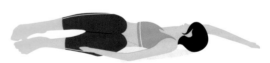

Hold up to 3 minutes and then come back to center.

92   7-DAY JUMPSTART PROGRAM

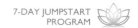

Savasana

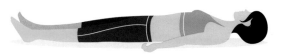

Lie down on your back, your legs outstretched in front of you. Arms stretched by your sides, palms facing up. Take two deep breaths in and out through the nose and release with a long sigh. Allow yourself to melt releasing any tension. All muscles should be relaxed, including the muscles in your face. If your mind begins to wander, bring your awareness on your breath. Stay here until you are ready to sleep or allow yourself to drift into sleep from savasana.

Deep Breathing

Stress often begins in our mind. If we can learn to quiet what we think, we can learn to control and reduce the stress we are experiencing. Our breathing has the power to do both. By bringing our awareness to our breathing, we can slow it down, which in turn slows down our heart rate, blood pressure and brings us an overall sense of peace and calm. Intentional deep breathing will calm the body and the mind and can prevent the activation of your sympathetic nervous system.

3 Deep Breaths Exercise

This exercise is SIMPLE! The next time you are feeling any anxiety creeping up, close your eyes and take three deep cleansing breaths. Slowly inhale through your nose, and slowly exhale with a long, sigh through your mouth.

When finished with your three breaths, keep your eyes closed until you find a natural rhythm, steady pace of breathing. Notice how you feel in the moment.

Meditate

Another fantastic way to de-stress and have more restful sleep is to meditate. Meditation has shown to decrease stress and anxiety, as well as bring a healthy balance to your body. You can easily meditate on your own. Follow a guided meditation or one of these simple, meditations below:

Click below to follow one of my powerful, guided meditations:

www.7dayjs.com/program

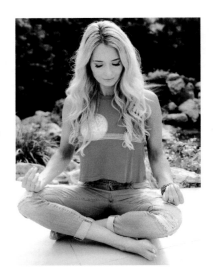

Body Scan Meditation

Find a comfortable seated position or lay down in savasana. If you are ready to go to sleep, you can also do this laying in your bed. Close your eyes. Take a deep breath in and out through the nose, and release with a long, audible sigh. Find a steady pace of breathing in and out through your nose, keep your focus on your breathing. Once you fall into a natural rhythm, do a full body scan, beginning from the top of your head and slowly traveling all the way down your body, to your eyes, your nose, your mouth, down both arms, to your belly, slowly down your legs and to the bottom of your feet and then very slowly, all the way back again.

Do this mindfully, and slowly, pausing at each section of your body sending calming energy. You can repeat multiple times until you begin to feel sleepy and allow yourself to drift into a restful sleep.

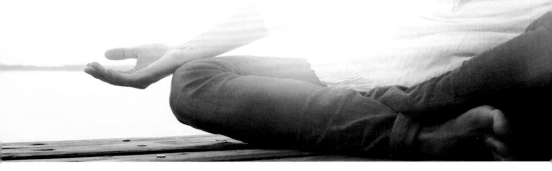

White Light Meditation

This meditation is very similar to the Body Scan Meditation, but we will visualize a bright white light. Find a comfortable seated position or lay down in savasana. If you are ready to go to sleep, you can also do this laying in your bed. Close your eyes. Take two deep breaths in and out through the nose, and release with a long, audible sigh. Find a steady pace of breathing in and out through your nose, keep your focus on your breathing. Once you fall into a natural rhythm, imagine a bright white light entering your body through the crown of your head. This light holds calming and peaceful energy. Slowly visualize the white light traveling down your body, sending this grounding energy to every cell in your body.

The light moves like a slow wave from the crown of your head, down your torso, down the arms, the fingertips and then all the way down both legs to the bottoms of your toes. Once this light fills your body, connect to the peaceful energy. As you inhale, imagine the light getting brighter and with each exhale you will experience more calmness and grounding. Visualize the light traveling all the way up the body and back out through the crown of your head. You can repeat multiple times until you begin to feel sleepy and allow yourself to drift into a restful sleep.

Eating Organic

What is organic food?

Organic food is food that is free of harmful pesticides or toxins that are typically used in conventional farming to protect crops from insects. We encounter many toxins in the air, water, personal care products and also in our food on a daily basis. These toxins are foreign to our bodies and can thus cause an inflammatory response when ingested regularly.

In a perfect world, we would eat 100% organic. But in our modern day, fast paced lifestyle this is not always possible and, we all know it can be expensive! I wanted to share a great resource with you that can support you in eating organic on a budget! This chart below is created yearly by the Environmental Working Group.

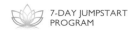

They list the "Dirty Dozen" which are the top 12 foods that contain the most amount of toxins that you should always buy organic, and they also offer the "Clean Fifteen" which are 15 foods that are safe to buy conventional. The clean fifteen typically have an outer shell or barrier that protects the food from the outside world so you can save money and purchase these foods even if they are not organic.

Clean 15 and Dirty Dozen

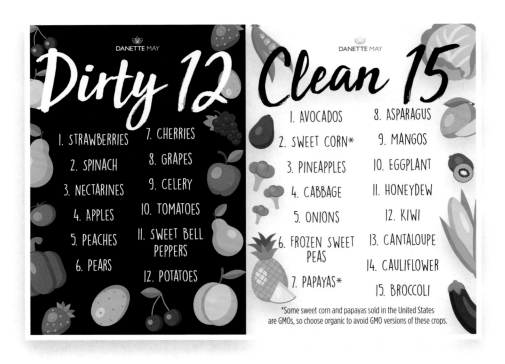

DANETTE MAY

Dirty 12

1. STRAWBERRIES
2. SPINACH
3. NECTARINES
4. APPLES
5. PEACHES
6. PEARS
7. CHERRIES
8. GRAPES
9. CELERY
10. TOMATOES
11. SWEET BELL PEPPERS
12. POTATOES

DANETTE MAY

Clean 15

1. AVOCADOS
2. SWEET CORN*
3. PINEAPPLES
4. CABBAGE
5. ONIONS
6. FROZEN SWEET PEAS
7. PAPAYAS*
8. ASPARAGUS
9. MANGOS
10. EGGPLANT
11. HONEYDEW
12. KIWI
13. CANTALOUPE
14. CAULIFLOWER
15. BROCCOLI

*Some sweet corn and papayas sold in the United States are GMOs, so choose organic to avoid GMO versions of these crops.

www.ewg.org

Congratulations!

Congratulations, you did it! You have stepped into the beginning of ultimate health and happiness by following this plan. The 7-Day Jumpstart was designed to get you started on the journey toward living a healthy and balanced lifestyle!

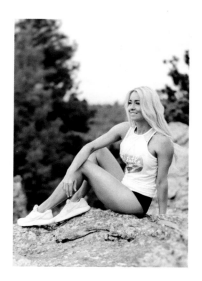

I have much more to share with you, and I want you to continue to be a part of my community and experience a deeper mind and body transformation.

I would personally like to invite you to join my 30 Day Challenge! The 30 Day Challenge is where you will progress further by receiving new workouts, delicious recipes, and powerful meditations. You will have all the tools you need to continue this healthy lifestyle and achieve your goals. I look forward to seeing you in my 30 day challenge!

www.DanetteMay.com/start30dc

Love,

Danette

Notes

7-DAY JUMPSTART
PROGRAM

Notes

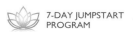

Recommended Resources

Upgrade To The 30 Day Challenge

This 30 Day Challenge is like no other! I'll show you how to LOOK and FEEL sexy and build your inner confidence, all without hunger, counting calories, or impossibly long workouts. Used by hundreds of thousands of women, you'll join an amazing community all getting guaranteed results in 30 days!

Visit www.DanetteMay.com/start30dc for more details.

Experience Superfood Healing Chocolate

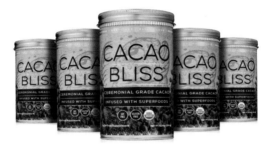

Cacao Bliss is an exclusive blend of raw Peruvian cacao powder infused with high-powered superfoods designed to beat your cravings and give your body the nutrients it needs to keep you healthy, trim, and energized.
Its rich, decadent flavor and healing ingredients make it a one-of-a-kind treat you'll enjoy daily.

Visit www.DanetteMay.com/7daycacao for more details.